Formulas for the
Apocalypse and Beyond
Shelter and Food edition

Formulas for the Apocalypse and Beyond
Shelter and Food edition

by
Matthew P. Camacho

To My Wife and Kids,
You Mean The World To Me

Acknowledgement

To declare that I wrote this book is like telling a concert conductor that they invented music. No, a better method would really to look at it as I have compiled these formulas so that is can seen in one place when there is no internet, no Siri and no Google. I did not create fire or develop boiling water I just did the leg work to help everyone in case the day people need to stand up again with knowledge that has been passed down through the ages. We will also keep it light and varied. If the world has come to an end this pocket of formulas to help you be creative in rebuilding a life and society.

Table of Contents

The Base

KISS

While these are formulas to help with your world and help you deal with it I will give you the first great Formula to apply to all the others. KISS, Keep it Simple Stupid. You have survived this long do not get to crazy use the formulas in the best methods you can to stay alive. If you are a minor reading and it is not the end of the world Please get a sane and responsible adult to assist you in any of these formulas.

FIRE

Let's start at the begging. Fire this
will allow you to
cook, work at night
and make water
safer. Now look to

$$E =. \frac{hc}{\lambda}$$

the right of the page. Do not worry
we will not use this formula. It is
just fun joke for a few smart people
(who are not me). Look on the next
page and see the fire diagram. No it
is not cheating it is a diagram but is
the formula to starting your new
civilization. There are some hints
in each of these.

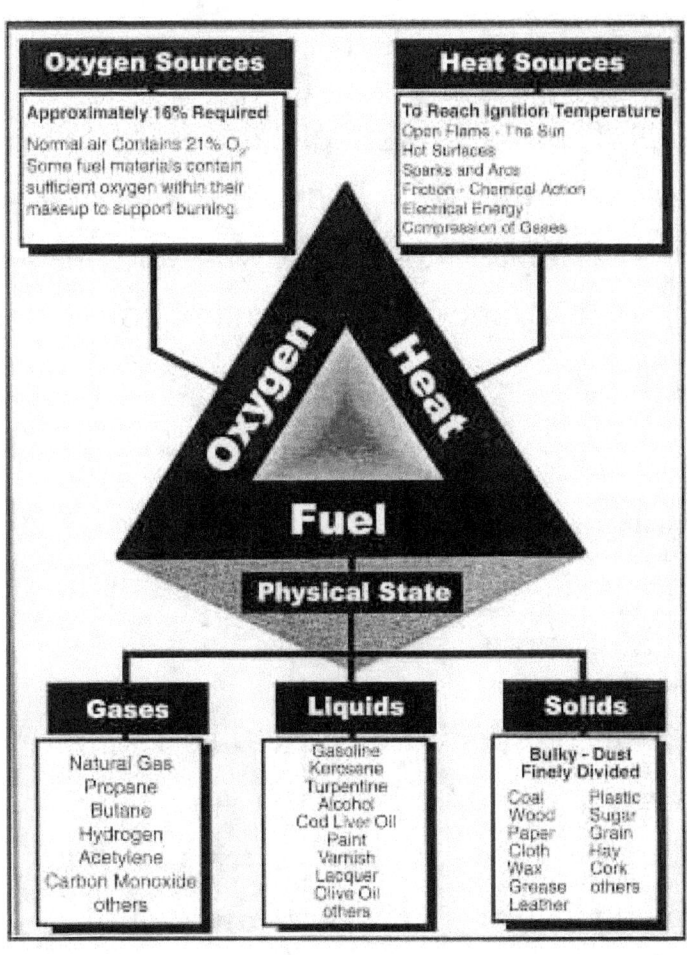

Oxygen Sources

Approximately 16% Required

Normal air Contains 21% O₂
Some fuel materials contain
sufficient oxygen within their
makeup to support burning

Heat Sources

To Reach Ignition Temperature
Open Flame - The Sun
Hot Surfaces
Sparks and Arcs
Friction - Chemical Action
Electrical Energy
Compression of Gases

Oxygen

Heat

Fuel

Physical State

Gases

Natural Gas
Propane
Butane
Hydrogen
Acetylene
Carbon Monoxide
others

Liquids

Gasoline
Kerosene
Turpentine
Alcohol
Cod Liver Oil
Paint
Varnish
Lacquer
Olive Oil
others

Solids

Bulky - Dust
Finely Divided

Coal   Plastic
Wood   Sugar
Paper   Grain
Cloth   Hay
Wax   Cork
Grease   others
Leather

Human Bodies Levels

There are some simple formulas to know about your body. If your fit bit or smart phone is down you can look at a clock for 15 sec and count your pulse. Then times it by 4.

BPM=X4, X is your count. You do not need to freak out about the decimals when doing your math it will just raise your heart rate.

Your temperature varies how and where you take it. Also your body can be .6 c or 1 f higher just by being you. Here is a simple reference to how your temp can change depending on method.

- **Orally.** Temperature can be taken by mouth using either the classic glass thermometer, or the more modern digital thermometers that use an electronic probe to measure body temperature.

- **Rectally.** Temperatures taken rectally (using a glass or digital thermometer) tend to be 0.5 to 0.7 degrees F higher than when taken by mouth.

- **Axillary.** Temperatures can be taken under the arm using a glass or digital thermometer. Temperatures taken by this route tend to be 0.3 to 0.4

degrees F lower than those temperatures taken by mouth.

- **By ear.** A special thermometer can quickly measure the temperature of the ear drum, which reflects the body's core temperature (the temperature of the internal organs).

- **By skin.** A special thermometer can quickly measure the temperature of the skin on the forehead.

Body temperature may be abnormal due to fever (high temperature) or hypothermia (low temperature). A fever is indicated when body temperature rises about one degree or more over the normal temperature of 98.6 degrees Fahrenheit, according to the American Academy of Family Physicians. Hypothermia is defined as a drop in body temperature below 95 degrees Fahrenheit.

CPR

It is highly suggested that you would learn CPR before the Apocalypse. Well it does change time to time on what the exact procedure there is very much some sound advice. CPR alone is unlikely to restart the heart. Its main purpose is to restore partial flow of oxygenated blood to the brain and heart.

An emergency procedure that combines chest compression often with artificial ventilation in an effort to manually preserve intact brain function until further measures are taken to restore spontaneous blood circulation and breathing in a person who is in cardiac arrest. It is indicated in those who are unresponsive with no breathing or abnormal breathing.

Compression-only (hands-only or cardio cerebral resuscitation) CPR is a technique that involves chest compressions without artificial ventilation. It is recommended as the method of choice for the untrained rescuer or those who are not proficient because it is easier to perform and instructions are easier to give over a phone. In adults with out-of-hospital cardiac arrest, compression-only CPR by the lay public has a higher success rate than standard CPR. The exceptions are cases of drowning, drug overdose and arrest in children.

As per the American Heart Association, the beat of the Bee Gees song "Stayin' Alive" provides an ideal rhythm in terms of beats per minute to use for hands-only CPR. One can also hum Queen's "Another One Bites The Dust", which is exactly 100 beats-per-minute and contains a memorable repeating drum pattern.

30Beat/2 breaths

Food

There are poets that can write volumes on food. There should be cooking books lying around with plenty on how to make food. But this is not a how to, but there is just a simple formula to know about your food. Canned foods really have a shelf life much longer than there expiration date. In 2012 there was canned corn examined from 1934. The sell by and sell by is not required by any law except for baby formula and some states require it for milk and meat. If come across can goods and the integrity of the can is still good the food should still be good for consumption. As for food to cook see the referred chart on the next page as the formula for your common cooked meats.

Meat	Internal Temp.	Centigrade
Fresh ground beef, veal, lamb, pork	160°F	71°C
Beef, veal, lamb roasts, steaks, chops: medium rare	145°F	63°C
Beef, veal, lamb roasts, steaks, chops: medium	160°F	71°C
Beef, veal, lamb roasts, steaks, chops: well done	170°F	77°C
Fresh pork roasts, steaks, chops: medium	160°F	71°C
Fresh pork roasts, steaks, chops: well done	170°F	77°C
Ham: cooked before eating	160°F	71°C
Ham: fully cooked, to reheat	140°F	60°C
Ground chicken/turkey	165° F	74°C
Whole chicken/turkey	180° F	82°C
Poultry breasts, roasts	170° F	77°C

The thermometer should be put in the meatiest part of the food.

Water

You need it besides you need it for every aspect of living many people do not know how to purify there water. You can to speed up the boiling and loose less while boiling is to cover it. **Be Warned** it can explode and steam is hotter than water. Boiling water is the most effective method of purifying it. To do so, you will need a heat source, such as a cooker or camping stove, and a vessel to hold the water.

According to the Washington State Department of Health and the United States Environmental Protection Agency, you should bring the water to boil and keep it rolling for one minute to purify it. At altitudes above one mile, 2,000 meters, you should increase the rolling time to three minutes. Other method s is 5 drops of bleach (non-perfume) per gallon of water.

Fish

Yes, Fish. Some people hate it and other love it. Fish can help rebuild a full society. Salt water fish is the safest and be eaten raw. Fresh water fish needs to be cooked. When cooking fish it should be cooked completely. Look there is a formula

:10 x 1"=cooked fish

That is 10 minutes for each inch of thickness. It should be flipped at the half way point. If the fish is thinner than a ½ inch it does not need to be flipped.

Tier 2

Shelter

You have most likely have had some form of shelter. There is not much that can be added to the shelter that should be laying around after the Big A has happened. But if you have been on the move and you can not go near former populated area(radiation, biohazard, zombies…) here is some helpful information on shelters.

Igloo

Diameter: Not to exceed 10 feet. Anything bigger would require a perfect dome, which is next to impossible to construct in the field.

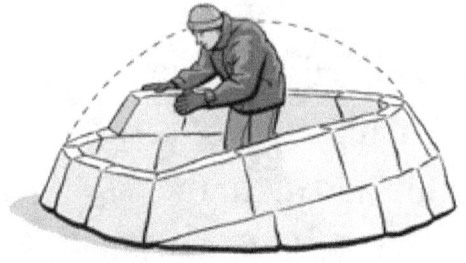

Mater ials: Top layers of dry powder won't work. Pack mounds of snow until they harden, or cut blocks of snow from the depth where your feet stop sinking.

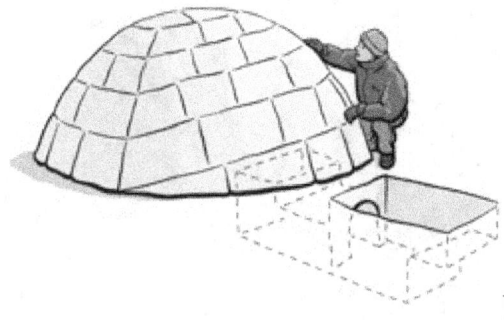

Entrance: Build a door in the ground, about 18 inches lower than the ground inside the igloo, and tunnel below the wall into the igloo. For proper ventilation, never seal or close the entrance.

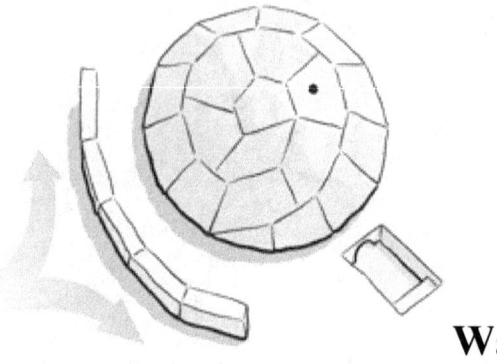

Walls:

Cut the blocks into a spiral layer, leaning one block against the next. Keep the interior wall smooth so moisture can run down the side of the wall, instead of dripping from the ceiling. Include a vent hole to allow for better circulation.

Earth Shelter

THE RIGHT SPOT

Choosing the best place to build a survival shelter is important. It should be in the driest spot you can find. Nothing sucks out body heat faster than wetness. If it isn't too cold, build a shelter on high ground. Breezes will help keep the bugs away, and you'll be easier to see if a search party passes nearby. If a cold wind is blowing, choose a spot sheltered by trees. But don't build in the bottom of deep valleys or ravines where cold air settles at night.

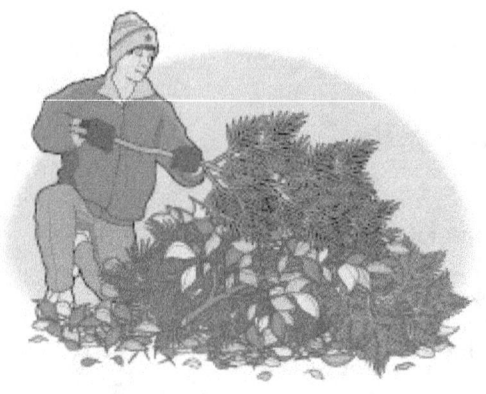

THE COCOON

If it's almost dark and you can hurriedly collect dry debris (leaves, pine needles, bark) from the forest floor, make a pile two or three feet high and longer than you are tall. When you burrow into the pile, you are in a natural sleeping bag that protects against heat loss.

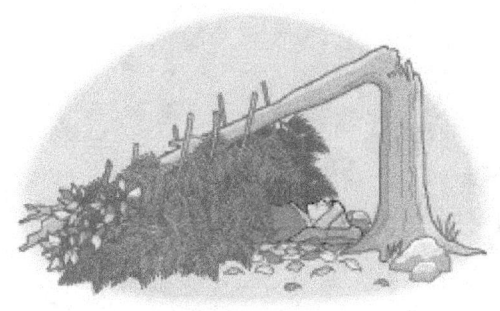

THE FALLEN TREE

The simplest shelter is a fallen tree that has enough room under it for you to crawl in. Lean branches against the windward side of the tree (so the wind is blowing into it and not against it) to make a wall. Make the wall thick enough to keep out wind. If you can build a fire on the open side of your shelter, the heat will help keep you warm.

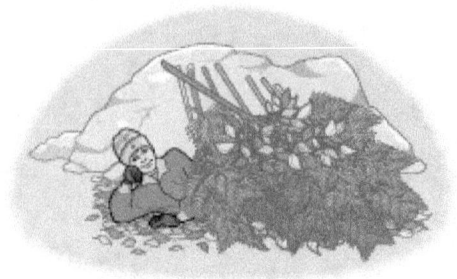

THE LEAN-TO

If you find a fallen tree without enough room under it, or a rock or a small overhang, you can build a simple lean-to. Start by leaning fallen limbs against the object, such as the top edge of an overhang, to create a wall. Lean the limbs at an angle to help shield rain. Cover the leaning limbs with leaves, boughs, pine needles, bark or whatever the forest offers. When you have built a thick wall, you can crawl underneath into your shelter. Remember to make your shelter no bigger than you need to fit you and anybody else with you. The bigger the space, the harder it is to keep warm.

You can also build a lean-to by placing one end of a long stick across a low limb of a tree and propping up the other end of the stick with two more sticks. Tie the ends of the sticks together with your boot laces or belt. Lean more sticks against the horizontal stick. Then pile leaves and other forest debris against the leaning sticks until you have a wall. Once again, a fire on the open side of the lean-to will add much heat to your "room."

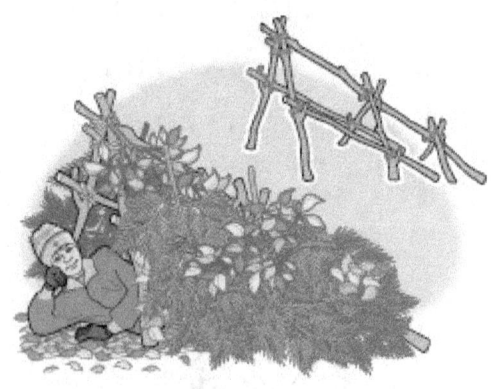

THE A-FRAME

If you can't make a lean-to, you can make an A-frame shelter. You'll need two sticks four or five feet long and one stick 10 to 12 feet long. Prop the two shorter sticks up in the shape of the letter A. Prop the

longer stick up at the top of the A.
Tie the three sticks together where
they meet. The three sticks will be
in the shape of an A-frame tent with
one end collapsed against the
ground. Now prop up more sticks
against the longer stick, and pile
forest debris against the sticks until
you have an insulated shelter open
at the high end.

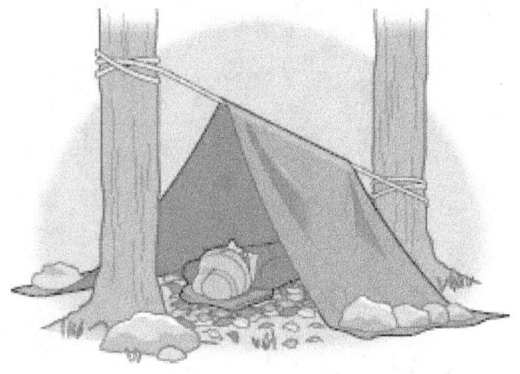

A TARP

When you have a tarp, sheet of plastic or Space Blanket with you, and some rope or cord, tie a line between two trees. Tie it low to the ground with just enough room for you to lie beneath. Stretch the tarp over the line. Place large rocks or logs on the ends of the tarp to hold it in place with the edges close to the ground. If it's snowing, tie the line off higher on the trees. Steeper walls will shed snow better. Now you have an emergency tent.

YOUR BED

Your shelter is not complete until you have made a bed to lie in. Dry leaves work well. Make your bed a little bigger than the space your body covers and at least eight inches thick. When you snuggle into it, you are ready for the unexpected night out.

BAD PLACES TO BUILD A SHELTER

1. Anywhere the ground is damp.

2. On mountaintops and open ridges where you are exposed to cold wind.

3. In the bottom of narrow valleys where cold collects at night.

Your Crap

Yes, this section is about your crap. Your waist, you generate 1 to 2 pints per day plus a 1 lbs of crap. Depending on how long you will be staying in an area and how many people you need to really think this out.   You can also use existing toilet seats out there cover and feel better about your new accommodation.

THE CAT HOLE

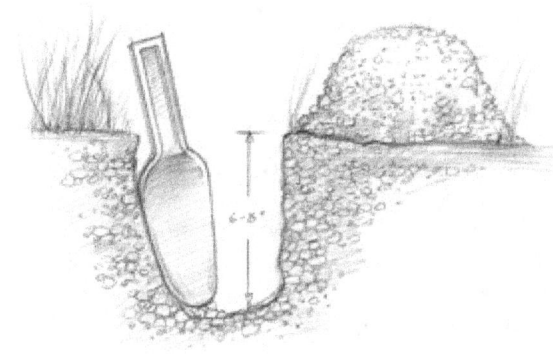

I n a short-term emergency, a few cat holes is all you need. Just take a garden trowel, a small shovel, or a post digger and make a hole about 6-8 inches deep and 4-6 inches in diameter. Do your business in the hole, wipe, throw the toilet paper (or leaves :)) in there too, and cover it up with the dirt you took out.

Although this is an easy method, here are a few rules you'll want to abide by:

- Place your cat-hole site is at least 200 feet from any source of water

- Don't dig in an area where water visibly flows (rain water run-off etc)

- Disperse the cat holes over a wide area if possible

- If possible, setup your cat hole in an area that gets a lot of sunlight (this will aid decomposition)

- Again, remember water runoff. Your every thought should be on preventing feces from reaching any water source — be it underground well water, your water table, rivers, lakes, springs, and creeks.

THE TRENCH LATRINE

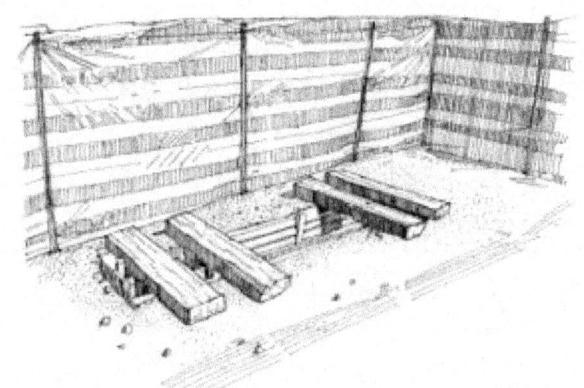

For a longer-term sanitation

solution, you'll want to build yourself a trench latrine.

A trench latrine is basically an oversized cat hole that is used multiple times. With the exception of dispersing it over a wide area, the same rules above apply to trench latrines as well.

The minimal recommended dimensions are around 1.5 feet (.45 m) wide x 1 foot (.3 m) deep and 2 feet (.6 m) long.

It's also recommended that you build some type of privacy partition. An emergency situation is stressful enough. You don't need to give anyone the added pressures of becoming a peep show. For example, a simple partition can be built with a few stakes in the ground with blankets, sheets or tarps stretched between them.

Since it is a multi-use station, you'll also want to prevent any flies and pests from coming into contact with the exposed excrement. To do this, after each use cover your business with some wood ash, quick lime, or a few inches of the dirt that came out of the ground when making the pit.

Conclusion:

Well you now have the basic formulas to ensure food (animal based) is cooked correctly, a shelter to live in and where to crap. This is very simple version on how does this all work and not as much on how to. You are a survivor and have lasted this long. Maybe you are on the run and you found this as you are thinking laying down your roots to build something more. Hopefully the house or library you found this book has more of the rest of the series to help you rebuild society and a way of life of people. Till then stay sharp.

References

How Long to Boil Water for Purification? |
USA Today. (n.d.). Retrieved from
http://traveltips.usatoday.com/long-
boil-water-purification-62933.html

How to build a survival shelter – Boys' Life
magazine. (n.d.). Retrieved from
http://boyslife.org/outdoors/3473/taking
-shelter/

Pins from organiceatingdaily.com on Pinterest.
(n.d.). Retrieved from
https://www.pinterest.com/source/organ
iceatingdaily.com